Skinny People Don't Understand

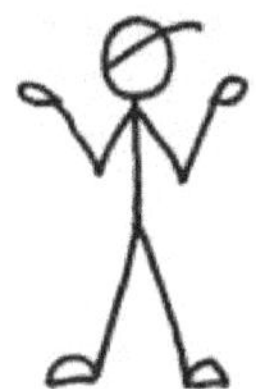

Michael J. Mendoza

ISBN: 1979424764
ISBN 13: 9781979424769
Library of Congress Control Number: 2017917250
CreateSpace Independent Publishing Platform
North Charleston, South Carolina

Table of Contents

Foreword

My GOAL IN life has been to become financially independent, spiritually fulfilled, emotionally stable, and physically fit.

I decided to write this book because I have come to understand that becoming physically fit has been my biggest challenge in life. Although I have never seen myself as morbidly obese, I am. I've always been a big guy. People close to me called me Mike. Then, because the name Mike was so popular, many started calling me Big Mike instead. I've always been cool with it—in fact, sometimes even proud of it. The problem is that over the years Big Mike got bigger. I have always had the gift of being able to consume extraordinary amounts of food. I'd take on food challenges in restaurants and be cheered when I won them. My association with food is very positive.

What finally triggered me to write this book is that all the advice I have ever received about losing weight has come from fit and skinny people. I begin this at a time in my life when I am age fifty-eight, weighing in at 301.9 pounds and having been stuck in this range of 300 to 310 for over ten years. I am five feet eleven. This is not my highest weight. I have been as high as 350, when sirens went off, but then I stopped gaining weight, and I have hovered where I am now for over ten years.

I have finally come to a conclusion: skinny people don't understand. It has become crystal clear to me that those of us who are grossly overweight are vastly different from those who are not.

I start this book now, not later, because I want to share the emotional and physical experience I am having and do not want to leave out or forget a single thing.

So for those of you who agree with me that skinny people don't understand, let's live this together. And for those of you *skinny people* who read this book, I hope you can better understand we are very different from you. We want your body. We want to eat cheeseburgers and ice cream and fries and nachos and beer and wine and cheese and donuts and cake and chips and pizza and not gain weight! We want to be able to run with the wind, but to curl up and have popcorn and other snacks while we look at fit people on TV is way more desirable.

I'm one week into this new program, hating what I'm eating. I'm in massive pain from the high-impact exercise. My wife says I'm cranky, and really, it's way beyond cranky.

I will succeed for one reason: I have decided to!

Whom is this book for?

- If you are like me and have always been overweight, this book is for you.
- If you have been on more than one diet plan and not had success, this book is for you.
- If you go to the gym and have been working out for years but you stay about the same weight, this book is for you.
- If you have successfully lost hundreds of pounds over your lifetime but still weigh the same or more, this book is for you.
- If you are depressed about your weight or your health as a result of your weight, this book is for you.
- If you are fit and never had a weight problem, but someone you truly care about has a weight problem, this book is also for you to help you understand what your loved one is dealing with.
- If you work in a fitness center and you are coaching struggling overweight clients, you need to read this to understand how we think. No, it is not logical!

Whom is this book NOT for?

- If you are fit and everyone around you is fit, this book is not for you.

Acknowledgements

First and foremost, I must thank my wife, Susie, for being the most incredible, supportive partner a man can have. Susie is doing this with me. She has set the same initial goal I have set of sixty pounds. *I am going to take care of myself for you, as I know you are going to take care of yourself for me.*

Second, I want to thank a couple of my mentors: Hector La Marque for his constant belief in me, Michael Gerber for planting in my brain the seed about transforming myself, and Steven Siebold for helping me with mental toughness. And finally, John Maxwell, for those words of wisdom in the first paragraph.

Finally, I want to thank all my cheerleaders on social media. I love you guys. And I can't leave out the over-the-top positive people at the boot camp I attended in my local area. I hate you and love you!

Chapter 1

The Start

DID I START here and now? Not really. I've started so many times. I've committed so many times. I've promised myself I'm going to do this so many times. I've voiced it loudly to people so many times. I've taken magic pills, potions, shakes, and almost every kind of quick fix out there. I've done low carb, no carb, and special prepared meals. I've done Nutrisystem, Jenny Craig, and Weight Watchers. I've had gym memberships and gone, stopped, and gone again. I've altered my eating habits, tricking myself into believing I was making progress.

Back in 1997, I was told by the doctor I had prediabetes. I had high levels of protein in my urine. But I felt fine. What do the doctors know? My condition gradually worsened, and later I was diagnosed with sleep apnea, in 1999. Rear-ending a couple of cars because I had just fallen asleep told me that something was wrong. None of this was sudden. It was just the effect of me not paying attention to my body. Maybe I should really get serious! So I did. A week or two later, I was back to the old me. Food has been my biggest happiness in life. It is the ultimate comfort. Yes, skinny people, you are going to have a great deal of trouble understanding this, but welcome to my world. I would go to the gym, sweat a bunch, but continue the same eating habits after a week or two.

The body is incredible. The abuse it can take is amazing. But it will reach a point where it can't continue to operate at those levels anymore. I once read that in life, you will always pay a price. You'll pay up front, along the way, or at the back end, but you will pay. I knew this, but for some reason I always thought I had plenty of time. When I was ready, I could always correct this.

Years have passed, and it's now 2011. I go into the doctor's office because I have sore knees as a result of running with my son. I haven't run in maybe twenty years. My weight is now over 345. Aside from my knees, I feel great. After ordering x-rays, the doctor tells me I don't really have a knee problem. What I have is a weight problem. Nonsense! It's the same me, Big Mike. I've just come back from a cruise to Mexico, and I have to pee every hour. I can't understand why I am so out of control. Must be what I'm eating.

The doctor says, "Mr. Mendoza, I want to order some blood studies. It's been quite a while." My blood pressure is extremely high, but I conclude I'm just nervous. OK, let's do the blood work. Three days later the doctor calls me and says I need to go in immediately. Oh, crap! Do I have cancer or something?

I go back in and now have to face something that makes no sense to me: my doctor tells me I am diabetic. I have high blood pressure, high cholesterol, high triglycerides, and extremely large amounts of protein in my urine. In fact, my doctor says, she can't believe I haven't had a stroke because my numbers are so high. Immediately, I am put on a whole bunch of medications and told I have to make changes in my life. Now scared, I immediately start to make changes. My numbers start coming down, and I drop forty pounds. I struggle because I hit a plateau. My numbers look good because of medication. Although I now need the medication to keep my numbers in control, my weight loss continues to be a struggle. I again revert to the old me but have become satisfied with my new weight. I have gone from a 48-inch waist to a 46-inch waist, from 4XL shirts to 3XL. I know I'm not where I need to be, but I justify and stay at this level.

Several years pass, and I change insurance, which causes me to change doctors. My new doctor sort of starts over. He says my numbers aren't terribly awful. I cross into age fifty-one, and he orders the dreaded colonoscopy. This is an age-reality check. I get through that OK, thank God. But the doctor says to me, at age fifty-two, "The quality of your life after age sixty will depend on your choices from here to there." That sticks with me. I know I have to do something or life is really going to suck, and sixty is approaching fast. So how does that affect me? Not much. I go to the gym more, but that's about it. Then I go to Weight Watchers. I really try, together with my wife. She and I start doing really well, and then I stop. Then she stops, and time passes.

My doctor sends me to a kidney doctor just to make sure there is no damage occurring to my kidneys. New tests are ordered. My numbers are not good. My medications are all increased. My blood pressure is too high, my triglycerides too high, my A1C too high, and my cholesterol too high. My weight, for sure, is way too high. But there's no kidney damage. With a change in medications and a little more awareness, I bring myself back under control, but I dread every new blood test. I am stressing as I approach my three-month visit. Why? Because deep down I don't want to change, even though I know I must. I read self-help books (again, written by skinny people), which motivate me for a moment. I tell myself, "You can do it, Mike!" But I don't make enough of a change to really matter. I change just enough to keep my testing in an OK, acceptable range for the doctor.

Then, while in Seattle, I see an infomercial. A doctor talks about disease, diabetes, and cancer and explains how our nutrition cures everything, including obesity. We order the DVDs, books, and everything that is offered. And off we go into a new eating regimen. It is July 2, 2012. My weight is 306.7. Eating a plant-based diet is difficult for me. Shifting away from cow's milk to almond milk is also very difficult mentally. But I'm committed. By July 26, factoring in one cheat day, I am at 288.2. Amazing! Not really, but I am making progress. Then I go on vacation. I come back and am 297.2. We start again because my wife is committed with me, but I know I give her grief. By September 7, I reach a new low: 286.9. My clothes are a little looser. I'm getting compliments. I have supportive friends, and everyone that is skinny wants to give me pointers. Well, that's it. I believe the hype and lose the discipline. I fall off the wagon and go back to the same old me.

So I get frustrated again, but not really, because it's much more the doctor threatening me than anything else that drives me to re-focus on weight loss. I restart on July 7, 2014. I weigh 306. By July 9, only two days later, I'm down to a whopping 302. Then I stop monitoring. That is an exciting restart. I am going to the gym two, three, sometimes four times a week. What have I learned? Altering what I eat will have a positive effect. So why don't I just do it?

For forty years of my life, that question of just staying focused on eating correctly has entered my head, lingered for a bit, then I get off track. I lose focus on what I'm eating and begin to justify eating the wrong things. I'm excited and motivated in every other area of my life, but it just doesn't happen when it comes to my weight. My knees hurt, but only occasionally. Otherwise I have learned how to scramble and keep my numbers within acceptable ranges so the doctors don't get angry.

July 2014, I injure my left ankle. I don't think much of it, but I'm now limping and waiting for it to get better. I alter my walk because of the pain. I buy an ankle brace and wait and wait. Finally, after six months, I go to the doctor. After x-rays and an MRI, I am told I've crushed the cartilage in my left ankle. There is no fix. I'll be fitted for an ankle brace and will probably have to wear it the rest of my life.

So with two sore knees, a problem with my ankle, type 2 diabetes, high cholesterol, high triglycerides, sleep apnea, and high blood pressure, I ask myself, "What's it going to take, Mike Mendoza?" I have mental arguments with myself all the time but never make a real change. I think if I just commit to losing weight, maybe I can fix all this. It seems like such an easy choice. But because I'm living in my body, it has never been an easy choice. Simple, yes. Logical, yes. Obvious, of course. But never easy. I am now again facing the battle I know I should have tackled so many times in my past and failed. This is the life of an obese person that skinny people just don't understand. It's like being broke, living paycheck to paycheck. I teach people how to change being broke, but most won't. It doesn't make sense to me. Why would you want to stay broke? I suppose it's just the same thing with a different issue.

We get comfortable. We get comfortable being overweight. We can buy bigger clothes. We can get stretch waistbands. Even sweatpants are made in sizes 2XL, 3XL, 4XL. Why do they make sweatpants so big? Not because we are going to work out and sweat, but because they are comfortable. Why are stretch bands added to pants? To give us the illusion we are still the same waist size, even though we are two to three inches bigger so we can feel more comfortable.

Chapter 2

Decision Time

My wife, Susie, gets solicited to join this boot camp. She tells me about it, and I tell her I'll support her. Then she goes to a meeting and tells me more. I am intrigued with their system and decide to go back with her. I know I need to do something, and this sounds different as well as challenging.

I make a decision: I'm going to do this. The initial goal is to lose twenty pounds in six weeks. I know I can do better than that if I stick to it. I decide I don't just want to lose twenty pounds; I want to lose sixty pounds, putting me at 240. This has been my goal weight for over thirty years. (They would like me to lose 110 pounds. Nice goal, but not possible for me to envision as realistic at this stage of my life.) I am setting this goal to be achieved in twelve to eighteen weeks. Susie sets the same goal of sixty pounds in eighteen weeks. That's three challenges. These are aggressive goals, but my mind tells me they are realistic.

We are given our nutrition plan. We are told we must follow it exactly. Every page of our booklet says FTDI (follow the damn instructions). We are told we must show up for a one-hour workout five times a week. We will weigh in the following Monday. Knowing this is my last weekend of freedom, I am going to eat everything I want before I can't ever again. Well, that's how I view it. Yes, I have an eating disorder, and I admit it.

As crazy as it sounds, rather than being scared or miserable or dreading the start, I'm excited about getting started. I'm allowing only positive thoughts to enter my brain. What will I look like sixty pounds lighter than I am now? What will Susie look like sixty pounds lighter? What an adventure we are heading on.

I tell Susie that once we have lost this weight, as a reward, we are going to empty our closets, donate all our clothes, and go shopping for new clothes.

I think, "Wow, I can shop in normal stores, not just those for large people." Skinny people don't understand this either. They can just walk into Macy's and buy something to wear. Not me, not ever. I've gone from 4XL to 3XL to now 2XL, and sometimes I get lucky somewhere and find something that might fit. But everyone has XL! My waist has gone from 48 with a stretch band to 46 and has stuck at 44, if I have that stretchy waistband—which really means I never left 46, but I can believe what I need to believe.

I also realize that after losing this weight, I will not have pain in my knees. In fact, I might even have no pain in my ankle. I can eliminate my medications. Maybe I won't have sleep apnea any longer and can get rid of my CPAP.

This is all very exciting. But deep in the back of my brain, I'm saying, "You know this isn't going to be easy. You know temptation is going to be all over the place."

I go back and revisit my other documented attempts at losing weight, the starts and the quits. If I break that twenty-pound mark, it will be my best attempt ever. Wait, let's rephrase that! *When* I break that twenty-pound mark, I will be entering uncharted territory. Not only will I do that, but I will do it in three weeks. I will FTDI. This is not going to be hard! I have an in-writing game plan. I know it will work. I know the only thing stopping me is me. I know the outcome is going to be amazing. I know I will be accountable to everyone because I will be posting my progress on Facebook every day I check in for my workout and every week for my weigh-in. I am not a quitter!

Week 1 begins! I weigh in at 301.9. It's not my highest weight in this yo-yo life I live. It's actually about my average for the last seven years, after coming off my real high of 350.

Starting my first workout, I could never have imagined what was going to take place. I don't wear an ankle brace, because in my past workouts, my ankle was annoying but didn't really hurt that much. The instructor says, "Jumping jacks." Sure, this is simple enough—until I try to *jump*. My mind knows what is supposed to happen, but my body laughs and says, "Uh, I don't jump. Sorry." I can't do one jumping jack. My ankle and knees will not allow this motion to take place. OMG, I'm exhausted, and we are just at the warmup.

This one-hour workout is not like anything I have ever experienced in my life. I feel as if my heart is going to blow out of my chest. I never realized an hour could be so long. There are no clocks anywhere. I have no idea how much time has lapsed. I just know I am on the verge of passing out. The trainer is so positive, and I am so destroyed. Today is the first time I can say this is what a real workout is, and I don't like it. I am saturated with sweat. I am dizzy and somewhat disoriented. We are told we will get used to it. It's like this for everyone the first week. I have entered the challenge of my life. We are in a mixed group of challengers and veterans, and it's really easy to tell who's who. I look at the veterans, and they don't look as I feel. I'm one click away from dying, and a bunch of these people look as if they can go another round.

We stretch and then get together and do a cheer. Day 1 is over! Our head trainer is Tim. He's like a young Anthony Robbins. He's a great guy, but I'm way too exhausted to tell him. My mind and body are not in sync, and being asked multiple times, "Are you OK?" confirms to me what I really look like.

I do not feel I am capable of doing anything the rest of the day. Fortunately, I have nothing planned. I am not motivated to change that either. I just want to go to sleep. We have to eat six times a day. Three of those meals are protein shakes. Breakfast is steel-cut oatmeal, but we need a protein and a vegetable. Another option is egg whites with a vegetable, but we need a carb. There is no bread, grain, seeds, or nuts allowed, just steel-cut oatmeal. Brown rice is permissible, as well as quinoa. What the heck is quinoa? I don't know what it is, but I do know I don't like it, even though I have never tried it. Our vegetables are limited to broccoli, spinach, brussels sprouts, asparagus, celery, and kale. We can't have lettuce, tomatoes, or cabbage. No beans of any kind. No fruit of any kind. Our other allowable proteins are fish, preferably tilapia, very lean ground turkey or turkey breast, white-meat chicken, and nothing else. No oils, sauces, or dressings. We must also have a gallon of water a day. No dairy of any kind, and no alcohol, because it would affect our metabolism. Eating will no longer be fun.

It's the perfect plan for a diabetic with high blood pressure and high cholesterol. Although it sounds very limiting, I know I can do this, because Susie is doing it with me. This will be fun. This will be an adventure. Everything about it sounds right. We also choose to buy all the products from our training camp. It's not an obligation. I just like the convenience, and we know what we are purchasing is correct. We also buy the supplements that we are supposed to take in the morning and before bedtime.

Although I am unable to function like a normal human being my first day, I don't regret anything. We are following the meal plan, and I am not hungry. I'm making it through the day. So is Susie. We have a lot of adjustments to make, but we are committed to making this our priority.

I'm getting in my water and finish it with my last supplement and my regular medications. We know tomorrow we are back at it with a workout at nine in the morning. We also know we need to start with a shake before our workout. It was a mistake to start our first day with an empty stomach.

Day 2, being very aware of what I am going to face, I dress differently. I put on my ankle brace, prepared for the challenges of another intense workout. But I know what to expect.

Arriving better prepared and starting to stretch, I realize Tim isn't there. We have a different trainer, this little mousy-looking guy named Junior. He starts to explain what today is. It's not going to be the same routine. Oh, crap. I thought I was prepared. Then he yells, "To the wall!" and everyone runs out of the back of the gym to the far end of the parking lot wall. I haven't run in so many years my mind and body are not communicating. I can't run. What the heck?

My knees are killing me, but my ankle, thank God, isn't hurting, because of my ankle brace. But three hundred pounds pounding on these knees isn't a good thing. So, obviously, I finish dead last. People are starting their warmups, and I'm still trying to catch my breath. I'm dying here, and we really haven't even started yet.

Junior explains the circuits for the day. We begin our workout. So how does today feel? It feels as bad as yesterday. There is more pain. I'm huffing and puffing. I know I have to be strong. Part of me says, "You just started. You can't do this!" And then I think how things go in my financial services business. We recruit someone, and they punk out and quit in a day or in a week because of lack of belief. I know how I feel about that person. I can't be that person here. No way!

It's painful, I'm exhausted, but I have to keep doing this. It's part of the grind. I have to change something I have been unwilling to change all my life. Of course it's not going to be easy. It's not supposed to be easy.

Day 2 workout comes to an end. I didn't die. I'm still standing, but very dizzy and light-headed. I walk out the door and sit down for a bit in the waiting room and drink some water.

We go home, and it's time for breakfast. I decide to check my sugar levels. Expecting to see low numbers because of my diet, I am surprised. My sugar tests at 257! OMG, this is not good. I check my test strips and realize they are expired by two years. It must be that. I'm going to buy some new test strips, because there's no way that can be correct.

They say don't weigh yourself. But I need to see some progress—after all, I'm two days into this—but I hold off. I don't feel well all day, but I have an interview to do, so I have Susie prepare me a shake, I shower and change, and I'm on my way. I'm exhausted, and it's taking hours for me to recover. I have a meeting in the evening, and I have to be there. Be positive and excited. I take a nap before my meeting, and I need it.

Day 3: I can't stand it, so I weigh myself. The disappointment happens when I look down at the scale and see no results. I have a scale that goes to 299 pounds and is accurate. So when I stand on it and the reading is 0, that means 300 pounds—and that's where the needle is. I go downstairs and check my sugar levels and get a reading of 261. For sure these test strips are no good. I have my shake. I don't feel good, but we head out to our workout. Today is legs.

I go to get new test strips to retest my blood sugar, but unfortunately the numbers are just as bad as they were with the expired test strips. I don't know what's happening. Maybe my body is just going wacky. I'm feeling odd, but with what I'm eating and how I'm working out, which is harder than anything I have ever done in my life, I've got to have positive results, so I keep pushing.

Day 4: Whoopee! Positive movement. I guess my body has decided to release some weight, and five pounds have disappeared. This week has been challenging physically and mentally. Anyone my weight or considered morbidly obese should not start a program like this unless you can take a week off and adjust to all the changes. For me, I am fortunate I have my own business and have the flexibility to adjust my schedule. But for the most part, I just want to go back to sleep every day. This has never been me. I'm always on the go, full of energy. I'm still confused by my sugar levels, because they are not going down.

Day 5: Thank you, Lord. This technically ends our workout week. We have two rest days and begin again Sunday morning. Today's workout was just as hard, but I'm getting used to it. My body needs to repair, so these two days are much needed. We continue to FTDI, eating what we are allowed and drinking one gallon of water a day. I have two back-to-back all-day seminars I must attend, and I buy a food travel pack to have my prepared food, water, and shakes with me to last the entire two days I will be away. This is a new and unique experience for me. It's so much easier to get a burrito or cheeseburger than to go through this, but I can't. I'm committed to this, and Monday is my first weigh-in.

Day 6 is done, and I did it. FTDI! No cheat day, no bending the rules, and I can't wait for my weigh-in on Monday.

Day 7: Workout 5 is not as painful. I needed those rest days. I'm very limited in what I can do physically, and I need to modify many of the exercises, because I just can't do what these veterans do with ease. I can't do anything that requires jumping, because it kills my knees and ankle. Then there are other things I just don't want to do. I'm capable of planking, squats, deadlifts, curls, and non-jumping things, but at my body size, these are challenging.

Day 8: It's weigh-in day. Before heading out, I have my shake and check my sugar levels. They're still high, but Susie has done some research on the supplement we are taking at night. Turns out it has an ingredient that not only can affect blood sugar but also blocks the effectiveness of my diabetes medication. Oh, crap. I've been killing myself, so I stop this immediately. Thank God Susie was just as confused and started investigating contents on labels. They have had no impact on her, but for me, I was very fortunate nothing serious occurred.

I weigh in, and *bam*, I'm down to 288.3! That's a weight loss of 13.6 pounds in one week. I am so excited to have these results. I know I can do this! My workout is still tough, but I'm making it through without as much pain. What else is totally exciting is that my recovery time is much shorter. On my first week, I was wiped out most of the day. I just wanted to take a nap. Not now. I'm good to go after about an hour.

Day 8 is like a new beginning for me. I don't want another egg white, and even though it's been just one week, I have to mix up the nutrition plan but remain FTDI. Broccoli is really getting to me, and I like brussels sprouts once in a while but not multiple times a week. I can hang with this eating plan a little longer, but not the duration of six weeks.

This second week is not much different from the first, but I'm getting more familiar with what to expect. There's tons of support and a very positive environment. Susie is a great partner through this. She's having difficulty with her back, and her pain is starting to seem greater than mine, so I have to stop being such a weenie. As I work through week 2, I am looking forward to a break at the end of next week. I don't think it could have been better planned. We will be headed to South Coast Winery in Temecula, California, for a three-day, two-night stay. I can push myself, thinking of this getaway. But until then, I look forward to Thursday, when I get a two-day rest from my workouts.

TGIT! Yes, thank God it's Thursday! It's the final workout of the week, and I'm so excited I've made it another week. Back on Sunday and weigh-in on Monday. I don't seem to be progressing so much this week. I think the first week was that shedding of what is called water weight, so my expectation is not high for Monday. But we must FTDI and cannot deviate from our nutrition plan. Saturday is a birthday luncheon for my mother-in-law. She has asked for Cuban food, and being married to not only a beautiful Cuban woman, but one can cook authentic Cuban food, it should be no mystery as to why I remain fat?

Saturday arrives, and there is Cuban food. OMG, I have to get through this without totally losing it and falling off the wagon. Arroz con pollo (chicken with rice cooked in saffron) is on the menu, as well as platanitos maduros (fried very ripe plantains), and since Susie is a cake decorator, what else could there be for my ninety-three-year-old mother-in-law but an incredible cake? I feel as if the world were watching, and I tell myself, "Don't punish yourself. Chicken is OK. Just be careful with your portions. Taste the plantains. Don't pile them on as normal. Sing 'Happy Birthday' and have a small slice of cake. Tomorrow you will be back on FTDI and work out in the morning. Keep drinking your water, and you'll be OK."

Not feeling punished and instead enjoying this one meal isn't as bad as I thought it would be. I weigh in on Monday, and I'm at 285.1, with a loss of 3.2 pounds. Not great, but I didn't go backward.

We're starting week 3, and things are still physically challenging, but I know I just need to make it to Thursday, because Thursday afternoon we leave for the wineries. We can sleep in! Oh, how incredible that sounds. I can't tell you how much this little getaway means. I am so looking forward to it. I am burning the candle on both ends with my workouts, then working until late, then waking up early to begin my workouts again. I'm eating what I don't want to eat, because it's necessary to hit my expected goals. Susie is ordering these prepared meals for us. It's going to make things so much easier on her.

We start with the new meals, and great news: Susie loves them. There's only one problem: I don't. As we try the different selections, the result is I like only one entree, the turkey meatballs. So after this one-week test, it's not likely we will be reordering.

I am eating the food but really struggling with it. I just keep looking forward: just get to Thursday. At the same time, we are having an incredible month in our business—in fact, one of the best in over five years. I am working like a dog this week, but Thursday is coming. I am committed to staying FTDI through Thursday night, and even though we are going out, we are going to do FTDI—with one exception. When I reserved this room, I ordered chocolate-covered strawberries and champagne for Susie upon our arrival. This was way before we committed to the camp. So although this is not in our plan, we are going to enjoy it without feeling guilty. But Friday, all bets are off. I have conceded Friday to no limitations. I have a normal breakfast, a wine tasting, a moderate lunch, and an incredible dinner planned.

Needless to say, Susie and I have an absolutely incredible weekend. Everything is fantastic. The weather is incredible. The hotel room is equally incredible, with a vineyard off our patio. We are so incredibly blessed to be able to enjoy such a weekend. We return Saturday afternoon, and it's back to the plan. Oh, how much I want to stop at In-N-Out Burger on the way home. But the getaway is over, and that is not an option. We have a protein shake on the way home and plenty of water.

It's Sunday, fun day! Workout is at eight in the morning. Although I really was off the plan and could feel it in this workout, I am happy we did it. Even though we screwed up, I was not able to eat as I used to eat. I think my stomach has shrunk. I am happy and rested.

I know taking these breaks is probably not recommended, but I have to learn how to maintain my life during this transition and see how my body reacts.

One thing I'm not stopping is my water intake: one gallon a day minimum. Watch the sodium, and stay clear of unnecessary sugars. Try to focus on protein. Salads with no dressing. No bread, no potatoes—steer clear of carbs as much as possible.

CHAPTER 3

It's the Second Half

IT'S MONDAY, WEIGH-IN day and the official start of week 4, the second half of my challenge. I weigh in at 281.6, which is a loss of 5.5 pounds. Not only am I still on track, but I am now at the lowest weight I have been at in over fifteen years. I am even more excited, and I do not regret our getaway. It was perfectly planned at the halfway point.

I have a blood test coming up this week and a doctor's appointment next week. I'm expecting my A1C readings to be out of whack because of the changes and the supplements that were in effect killing me. I am so thankful Susie figured out the problem before something serious occurred.

This week I'm noticing the workouts are still just as challenging, but my recovery time is immediate. I get in the car, and I'm fine. I have energy and am ready for my breakfast, a shower, and the beginning of my work day.

Our financial services business is crazy. We had our best month last month and are ready to start a new one with a new contest for our team. Our winning team from last month will celebrate this Saturday by going to a go-kart indoor racetrack. This team is mega competitive, so this is going to be fun. They are all twenty-one and younger, and Susie and I are going to be racing with them. Then we're off to dinner with them all. We must stay focused this week because Saturday night is going to be a pizza party—pizza and beer. Well, it's something to look forward to. I just need to have that carrot to get me through the week. I'm feeling good. My ankle is being cooperative. My knees are still hurting bit, but I'm running.

Susie has found another way to get our meals. A local store has started preparing FTDI meals. We go together and visit the store. It's not very impressive but has an A rating. We order a week's worth of meals. Great news: Susie loves the meals. And guess what: so do I. We have found a part-time solution to our meal plan.

I am informed this week that my aunt on my father's side (his sister) has died and my father and stepmother will be coming to stay with us next week to visit and attend the funeral.

Also this week I decide to buy a new car. One, it's time, and two, hey, it's going to be a new me. What a better time to make such a decision?

This is a week of excitement. I'm excited about my new car. I'm excited about my progress at our boot camp, I'm excited about celebrating with our team winners and having my "cheat" meal this weekend. Although not under the best of circumstances, I'm also excited to see my dad and stepmom next week. They live in Sacramento, and we don't see them much.

There is no question I need to be mentally prepared to tackle this boot camp and stay focused, but having these positive distractions is actually helping me through this. I'm not dwelling on what I don't like or want to do but rather focusing on the exciting things that are continuously happening or going to happen.

I'm just keeping one foot in front of the other, a new day, then another, then another, and TGIT. Yes!

I have a Friday-morning accountability meeting for my business at seven, and tomorrow is Friday. I visit with my leaders after the meeting, which is always enjoyable.

Saturday is here. I have my protein shake and head to my first appointment, scheduled for ten o'clock. My day isn't too busy, and I'm looking forward to our team event tonight.

So what does tonight's go-kart racing have to do with anything? Well, everything. My competitive juices start flowing, and I want to win. Every one of these kids I beat is a feather in my cap. With my weight I'm not going to win on speed, because I am already at a huge disadvantage, but I can out-skill these kids. So we're off. First there's a qualifying round. I don't do so well, but now I'm going all out.

I'm passing one, then another. They are spinning out, and I'm pushing myself to the limit. And then I'm pushing to lap one of my guys, Tyler. He's trying to fight me off, but I'm coming, and I'm coming fast. We go around a turn, and I know I'm going to get him here. He spins out, and I can't avoid him, and T-bone his cart at full speed. Now I'm a little large for these carts, so I'm sitting a little awkwardly. At impact my lower body slides forward. Remember my ankle with crushed cartilage that was just feeling better with my weight loss? Well, this impact really does it in. When I get out of the cart, I know I really screwed it up. I had no business racing, but I did. They all wanted me to, and so did I. There are some things you just wish you could take back.

I show no hurt. We leave there and are off to pizza. I am in pain, so why not have a beer? Maybe it will help. Well, a second can only be better. And then I catch myself. *Stop!* Bring me some water. It was fun. I fell off the wagon for a minute but regrouped. Tomorrow is a new day, and my workout is at eight o'clock.

I put my ankle brace on in the morning. I am having trouble just walking. How am I going to work out? But I must. Just no running today. I must be FTDI and drink a bunch of water, and fortunately my body responds by keeping me in the toilet for my regressions. It's as if the body knows it was poisoned.

I arrive, stretch, and tell the trainer I can't run at all, so when everyone is running, I'm on the stationary bike. My body responds well, and I get through my workout. However, running isn't an option this week.

Each new day, working out is starting to become part of my normal routine. Each day may be different and always challenging, but this group of people we have surrounded ourselves with is fantastic. It's not just Susie and I; it's Susie and I and new supportive friends. Sure, there are some grumpy nonsocial ones, but overall, it's a great environment.

I started this boot camp on September 14, 2015, and FTDI is constantly being reinforced. I've messed up, but it's been all mental. It's clear that I'm going through a transformation in what I eat (mental) and how I work out (physical).

It is now October 12, 2015, and weigh-in day. My weight is 278.6. I am down 23.3 pounds, and I have crossed another threshold. Although I see the same person when I look in the mirror, I know that I am not. My clothes are all loose—in fact, so much so that I need new pants. Shirts that I didn't wear because they were too tight and uncomfortable now fit, and I have extra room. Tomorrow is a doctor visit.

October 13, I weigh in at the doctor at 278 pounds. My blood pressure is 124/70. I am so proud of myself, but the doctor isn't. Much to my surprise, my A1C is still very high. It's very confusing for me because I've lost so much weight. I changed the shakes and stopped all supplements—but apparently not in time to affect my A1C. But my doctor is seeing the fruits of my effort and wants me to come back in four months to be retested. My ultimate goal is to come off all medications. He believes I will be able to eliminate my high blood pressure medications on my next visit. As for the diabetes medications, he's not so sure. But we'll see.

Due to the death of my aunt, my dad and stepmother come to stay with us for five days. Susie and I must stay FTDI. They too have been great cheerleaders of ours. After the funeral, there is a luncheon, and we stay strong when choosing what we eat. On Saturday, we attend a charity dinner. Again, temptation is there, but we both continue making the right choices.

And then comes test number three: we treat everyone to Sunday brunch at Marie Callender's. It's my grandson's birthday, and he loves buffets. So we're off to minimize the damage we can cause to ourselves. Although I'm not 100 percent, I focus on staying around proteins and very minimal carbs. No desserts, and that is the toughest of all, but I know I have a weigh-in Monday.

So here we are, Monday morning, October 19, with just one more week to go. My goal was 30 pounds by the end of six weeks. I weigh in at 273.3. I have dropped another 5.3 pounds. Although I'm not at my goal weight, I know I can hit it. I still have another week to go!

I stay FTDI, but I am concerned. Although I don't feel constipated, I'm just not going. I continue to pee very frequently, but that's it. It's as though my body is completely consuming whatever I eat and producing no solid waste. How will this affect my final week of weight loss?

Friday is Susie's birthday. Her goal is to weigh out on Friday morning so she doesn't have to stress about what she eats for her birthday. My schedule will not allow me to share in this choice. She is struggling with the weight and goes on "talapigus": basically just tilapia and asparagus three times a day, and water. Then, on her final day, she has this dieters' tea. Off to the toilet she goes, over and over again. I have never seen her so stressed and driven to hit this twenty-pound weight-loss goal.

Susie has her weigh-in on Friday morning and hits her goal. She's actually lost a total of twenty-three pounds. I am so proud of her. Tonight we celebrate! We are going out to a Mexican steakhouse. OMG, I'm not weighed in yet, and I'm so close.

Do I control myself? Absolutely not! My willpower goes right out the window. But I tell myself this is one meal, not the end of the world. I still have Saturday to regroup and a Sunday-morning workout. Then there's that dieters' tea. The problem is I have a training for my representatives on Sunday night, and I must be careful with that tea. Susie says it takes four to five hours to kick in, so I go for it. I shouldn't feel anything until after nine o'clock.

I'm not going to weigh myself. My fate is in the tea. Nothing happens. Oh, crap (literally): there is none. My body is stuck. My weigh-in isn't until eleven thirty the next morning, but what do I do? I guess nothing, so we watch TV and then go to bed.

It's six in the morning, and there's an emergency trip to the toilet. The tea has decided to kick in, and it came with a vengeance. After two-plus hours of this joyous experience, I figure wherever I'm at is the best I can be.

October 26: It's weigh-in time, and it's amazing! I weigh in at 267.3, finishing with a loss of 34.6 pounds in six weeks. I am the biggest loser for our center! We now have a week off but have committed to another twenty-pound challenge. My personal goal is thirty pounds again.

CHAPTER 4

It's Break Time

CLOSING OUT THE month of October with our first-ever Halloween party, we tell ourselves we are going to work out on our own and be mindful of how we eat. Then, when we restart, we have a three-day getaway to the desert.

Break time was definitely a learning experience. Now we are not being held accountable. We are away from the group. We clearly know what we should be doing.

The day after weigh-in, I schedule a field trip with a couple of my guys. I take a shake with me and stay focused on my water. Overall it's a good day because I stay busy.

The next day I start early with a chamber meeting. What's there but donuts and coffee? I walk in with my water, and people notice my weight loss. There's no way I can eat a donut after telling them of my six-week experience.

I pick up Susie, and we decide to go to one of the unhealthiest places to eat breakfast. Susie and I have the day together, just running errands, and start absolutely the wrong way. Why? Because we are "rewarding" ourselves for doing such a great job. Then that night we take our son Mark out for his birthday. We head to a local Indian casino, and we all win money. Those are some astonishing odds broken. So we head to the most logical place for dinner: the buffet.

Again, left to my own devices, I mess up. I really go on a binge. It's as if I feel if I don't eat everything now, it will never be there again. Here again is something skinny people don't understand. We less-fat people are still just fat people who have lost some weight. It is clear six weeks hasn't changed too much mentally.

In addition, I never seem to find the time to work out on my own. I know what I'm doing isn't the right thing. I know my choices haven't been the best, but I think because I know I have a new challenge in a week, I will get myself back on track.

We head out the next day to Baja, California, just a day-trip, and we start off the morning the right way. After we cross the border, I make the call for lunch. "Let's go to Puerto Nuevo and have lobster for lunch." Susie says that sounds good to her, and we are off. The lunch is incredible. We sit with an ocean view and totally enjoy the time together. Just to be clear, lobster Puerto Nuevo style is deep fried—not FTDI at all. But what I have learned to do is to really enjoy the meal. I know it's not something that will be frequent in my life, so I want to take my time and take it all in. I have always eaten a lot, but I never consciously enjoyed these bad choices so much as I am enjoying them now.

After a great day shopping in Baja, we head for home. We get back on track for dinner, knowing we potentially have some more bad choices that we will be facing this weekend.

We do FTDI through Friday and Saturday morning. But it's now Halloween. We order the Taco Man for the party. I, of course, fall off the wagon again and regress to the old Mike. Even though I stay away from as many sugary treats as possible, I still make a ton of bad choices. I will say, however, I have a great time!

Sunday morning I buy everybody breakfast, and I continue with bad choices. Again, knowing I'm back on it tomorrow leads me to choose food I know is completely off limits for the next six weeks. But I also know there will be no weigh-in, because they are using my weigh-out numbers for the start.

This craziness is now over. It's Sunday night, and all must change. I have learned how much I lack discipline when I'm not held accountable. I've got a lot of work to do. I weigh myself at home and realize this one week I gained ten pounds.

I am so grateful I don't have to weigh in, and know I've got to get it together.

Chapter 5

Challenge #2

It's really good to be back. Susie and I both messed up, but I beat her because I *really* messed up. We start our new challenge determined to get it going in the right direction, but we know we have another getaway planned for the end of the week. I remember how excited I was about Thursdays. It is our last workout for the week. I can stay focused for the week knowing I just have to get to Thursday—especially this one, because we were headed to Palm Desert to stay in an incredible resort.

With four days of FTDI, we can pull this off. Workout 1 coming back is familiar but very challenging. But it isn't like day 1 of the first challenge. Each day I tell myself what a great getaway this is going to be. The workout days are so much easier to deal with. Although they are still very challenging, they aren't the same they were in the beginning. I do believe having done so many, I am able to handle them much better, and there is less of me to push around. I'm still trying to catch my breath; I'm still getting beat up. But I know what to expect. I'm not going to die.

Thursday has arrived. I know I'm still not at my original weigh-out weight, but I'm excited to enjoy the next three days. We are cautious with our Thursday eating. We have room service for breakfast and just sleep in. We spend a day shopping and then totally screw up our choices for lunch and dinner, especially dinner—so much so that I felt sick.

The following morning, we have room service again for breakfast, but just steel-cut oatmeal and coffee and a whole lot of water. We head back and know we have another workout Sunday morning.

Damn, it's weigh-in day, and I know I'm over. But I must weigh in. It's mandatory. Honestly, I totally forgot about having to do this, and the fear doesn't hit until I pull into the parking lot. I weigh in at 273.3. I am up and over my weigh-out by six pounds. Although it's not the end of the world, it is clear I still lack the discipline to maintain my weight loss.

Without question, those of us fighting this battle must understand we are not going to do this alone. Not only do we need the desire, but we need the accountability every week. So it's back at it. Like it or not, I must remain FTDI.

We have no travel plans for the remainder of this challenge, but there is Thanksgiving. I'm not looking at Thanksgiving as a day I alter what I eat. I'm going to mess up. I'm not going to kid myself; it's one of my favorite days of the year. As I watch the skinny people talk about alternatives like Tofurkey and I hear about all the healthy recipes they suggest, I concede. I will just work harder and not fool myself. This day will be like my getaway day. I am going to enjoy the food. I will not be FTDI that day. But I also know it can be only that day. Until then, stay on the plan!

I'm doing excellent this week! I'm feeling good, and after my workouts, although they're tough as always, I have excellent recovery time. I have conditioned my body to the point where I am totally recovered within thirty minutes.

My blood pressure has been great, and I decide to start checking my sugar levels again. My levels are actually on the low side. So for now I'm excited. The week goes by exactly as planned, and I stick to the plan. The problem I am having again, however, is constipation. I don't feel backed up, but nothing is happening. Fiber One bars have zero impact. Could there be something wrong? Is my body consuming everything and leaving behind no waste whatsoever?

I have a great wife! She is struggling with this challenge, and I feel so bad for her. I want her to have better success than I have. She is really getting frustrated because she has had to make up weight gain as well and now is not progressing. But I know I couldn't have done any of this without her help. She has got new recipes and is mixing up our meal plan. She's spicing up the food. These change-ups are helping tremendously.

I realize many of you reading this won't have that wife to do these things for you. I am so sorry for that. You will have a rougher go of it, because it takes time to prep these meals. My suggestion is to prep and plan as much as you can, maybe even purchase prepared meals. It's amazing how these are becoming available in many areas. We get meats from a company called Meats2U.com. I have no financial interest in this company, but their meats are great! They cost more, but if you're going to do this, taste is everything. They are pre-seasoned, FTDI friendly, and packaged in the correct portions. That's my plug for them.

It's Monday again. Now I am looking forward to my weigh-in. Yes, I have been checking, which is why I'm excited. My official weigh-in is 265.9! I have hit a new low. Although not on track, because of my gain, I am proud of myself because I now weigh less than I have in the last twenty years. These positive weigh-ins make it all so worth it.

I am a fat person wanting to be fit, wanting to be healthy, wanting to not have to take medications for high blood pressure, diabetes, and high cholesterol. I will always be that fat person, regardless of my weight loss. I think we must come to grips with this. It's always going to be a battle. I will never be a skinny person eating what I want and not gaining any noticeable weight.

But I can eliminate those medications. I can extend my life expectancy and improve the quality of my life. It feels good to weigh less! Yes, it does! These are all choices.

I need to give up many of those things I love to eat and replace them with foods I must eat. I love bread with butter. I love cheese. I love fatty, greasy foods. I love having salads submerged in blue cheese dressing with bacon. My favorite ice-cream flavor is rocky road; my next favorite is every other flavor produced. I love fruit pies and cream pies; in fact, if it has the word "pie" in it, I love it. A loaded baked potato with a thick juicy steak and sautéed mushrooms is heaven. My favorite fish is deep fried, and ribs, pork or beef, make me smile. Pastrami with chili fries or pizza and beer or wine and pasta—I'm excited. All these things are what got me in the predicament I'm in. Are they bad for me? Yes. Have I learned how to connect the word "moderation" with these foods? No.

I am not sure how the maintenance plan is going to go here. What I do know is I am not willing to give these things up. I need to learn how to integrate these things into my life without returning to the person I was. I'm thinking it will be trial and error. Maybe one bad day, maybe just one bad meal. My body will be my guide.

The most exciting thing I did this week was bag up all my old pants and belts, which were all way too large, and donate them. There is definitely less of me. Susie bought me some new pants that, although I'm not at my final weight or size, I had no choice but to buy. I had to find some pants that looked nice but were inexpensive. She got me four pairs for twenty dollars each. I'm telling you she's awesome! I still have some big clothes, but I know they are all on their way out. If I don't keep the big clothes, I know that will be a good guideline for the future if I get off track.

As a reward, I want to take Susie to get a new pair of designer jeans, one pair for me and one for her. Expensive, yes, but even our jeans are too big. I'm excited to be a new size. Even though I know this size will be temporary, we need to do this.

What's even more exciting is that people are following me on social media and cheering me and Susie on. Then we see people, and they say, "Wow!" When I see myself in the mirror, I don't see much change, but I know it's happening, based on other people's reactions and the clothes I'm wearing. This happy feeling must stay with me.

With this new week, I am checking my sugar levels more frequently. My numbers are low. Actually too low—I'm in the 60s. Even after a meal, I'm still below 100. Sometimes I feel a little jittery. I know this is because of my sugar. But I also know this is a good sign, because I am taking medication that may now be too strong for me. Yeah! I call my doctor and wait for a reply. Hopefully, we can cut back some of my meds.

Our last workout of the week is on Thursday. It's my favorite day because I get two days of rest. This workout turns out to be so intense. In fact I believe we have the hardest workout since we started. I am gasping for air but not panicking. I have discovered that part of my mistake in the first week happened because this was uncharted territory for me. That first week I was dying, but I was also panicking during my workout, which increased my anxiety. Now it's OK. No matter how hard it is, I know it's going to be over soon. I won't die. And I know when it's over, I'll feel great as soon as I get home.

It's Friday, and I have my weekly business accountability meeting. It starts at seven o'clock, and I usually go with my team to a local fast-food place that has virtually no good choices. I've messed up here before, and today is no different. I have a protein shake in the morning and then screw up with a breakfast burrito. Why? Because that's what fat people do. I have coffee with Splenda—and yes, I know it doesn't cancel out the burrito. I leave after our accountability meeting and head to another meeting. I'm out of water, so I stop at a minimart to buy a water. The problem is I also buy a giant Twix bar. Why do I do this? I know it's totally the wrong thing to do. I know it, I think it, and I get back in the car and eat it. I enjoy every bit of it! When I'm done, I ask myself, "Was it worth it?" I don't know the answer to that question. I do know I have no problem with low sugar levels today.

Although Saturday is a rest day for me, I have decided to go to my old gym and do some cardio. One reason is to pay myself back for the burrito and the Twix bar. I haven't been there in over two months, because I've been going to this boot camp. It'll be interesting to see how it goes. My intention as I write this is to really push myself. But for now, my day is over. A little TV, then bed.

Sunday begins with my technically "close-of-the-week" workout, since our weeks begin on Mondays. I'm glad I did the Saturday cardio. I'm thinking it may have to become a part of my routine. This second boot camp is not as easy a weight-loss experience as the first was. I have, however, lost a great deal of inches, which is showing in the clothes I am wearing. Because of the cardio, my workout doesn't really seem that difficult today. I do know my weigh-in tomorrow isn't going to be good, but it will not be a surprise.

It's Monday morning and time to weigh in and begin a new week. The date is November 23, and I stand on the scale. I weigh in at 261.2. We hear from the founder of our boot camp on a Facebook video that if we stay all protein, zero carbs, we can have a normal Thanksgiving feast. We get to eat all we want and anything we want for this one meal. We cannot deviate at all before or after this Thanksgiving feast. The trick is to stay all protein and keep up the workouts. Our camp is open Thanksgiving Day with three morning workouts. I can do this!

Thanksgiving morning we are there, ready for our workout. So are about a hundred people I've never seen before. It is a brutal workout, with half of us outside and the other half inside. After thirty minutes we switch and finish inside. There's been lots of running, and this has been killing my knees. More than ever I am in a great deal of pain. The last three days I have not slept well, because everything is hurting. I wake up to pee every two hours and face the pain.

Before starting my workout, I didn't think it would be possible. The pain I was feeling was everywhere. But for some strange reason, it goes away when I begin working out. Not totally, but I have gone from difficulty walking to completing the workout.

We come back and have a protein shake. I'm drinking these BCAs that were recommended. They have no sugars and have not affected my blood glucose levels, so they are working fine. They also are supposed to help a little with the soreness, as well as curb my appetite. I'm thinking this week has been so painful because I have been on zero carbs.

A little later I have a spinach omelet, staying only on protein. I will have about a two-hour window when I will be able to eat anything I want and put myself into a food coma, so all this will be worth it. That's the fun part about Thanksgiving. I can't wait!

The moment comes. I can eat like the old me. Everything is fair game. There are no limits. But after one plate, I'm done. I cannot eat any more. I love pumpkin pie, and now I can have as much as I want. I told Susie earlier to bake one just for me. What happens? I'm full, but I'm going to have some anyway. I eat it and wish somehow there were a way I could fit more. But I can't. The feasting is over. I wanted more of everything, but yet I didn't. There was no desire to eat more, because I was stuffed.

I sleep great. There's still pain, but nothing like the last few days. Tomorrow will be a day of rest from my workouts. But we do have to start putting up the

Christmas lights. Fortunately, I have two adult boys that I can still coerce into doing most of the work.

I manage to stay on track the whole day. Zero carbs for another two days to complete this process called carb cycling. I'm planning a cardio workout at my old gym, just like last week. It's low impact but very effective. I want this next weigh-in on Monday to have me back on track.

My cardio workout comes with ease. I hardly break a sweat. Twenty-five minutes on the elliptical, squats, and then twenty-five minutes on the bike, and I cannot get my heartbeat over 110, no matter how hard I push. I suppose this is a good thing. My recovery is immediate. So it's clear my health has improved as well as my endurance. I did gain about five pounds from Thanksgiving, but I'm drinking a lot of water and holding to no carbs until Monday. I'm feeling less pain and am ready for a return to boot camp on Sunday.

Sunday is here, and it's time for boot camp. I weigh in and still must drop five pounds by tomorrow, but I am confident if I stay on FTDI and keep up the water intake, I will be OK. Today's workout is a lot of cardio, which doesn't compare to what I did on my own yesterday. These are real workouts. Because my bootcamp is so intense and my old gym is just normal, I refer to my old gym as Camp Snoopy. There is clearly a difference, but I don't regret doing that extra cardio.

Monday morning, and it's weigh-in day. I feel great. There is no pain! Our bodies are incredible. I decide to weigh in after my workout. It's upper-body day, and we have Junior. Junior is very different from the other trainers, but I have grown to know him a little better. We had him Sunday as well. Junior and "running" are synonymous. His favorite phrase is "to the wall," and you know it's coming. He's a little less organized and structured, but you know the workout is going to be challenging. He has this evilness about him that is a part of his persona. Having different trainers and constantly changing routines is what makes this work. It has been an incredible experience. We finish, and it's time to weigh in. I weigh in at 259.7, a new low. I am still way behind, but I'm excited. My overall goal was 240, but for this challenge, I only have two weeks left. My final weigh-out will be on December 14. I must be at a minimum of 247.3.

Susie is frustrated. She has not deviated from FTDI but is not losing weight. She has noticeably lost inches, but her body has not lost weight in this challenge. I told her we are going to make a commitment to lose ten pounds each this week. In her case, if she doesn't do it, she will be disqualified. Although she says she's OK with it, I know it's devastating her. We have to do this together and give it our best shot.

CHAPTER 6

The Push to Complete Challenge #2

IT STARTED WITH a decision. We have had to separate our business lives and personal lives from our challenge lives. We started with a decision and commitment to do this in the first challenge, and now we need to push ourselves harder than ever in the second challenge. Deep down I know this challenge is going to be more difficult because we are transforming our bodies, and they may not be so willing to make this radical a change in such a short time span. But we know it can be done, because it has been done repeatedly before us.

In my business it becomes stressful at month end. We are never where we want to be and must push at the end of the month to get in as much as we can. Today is November 30, and it's month end for our business. We are going to have to treat this next week in our challenge as if it's month end every day for the next seven days. Each day we must tell ourselves, "Just one more day." Now I know we can't expect to live our lives this way, but for the time being, we must bring our weight down. Maintaining our weight will be a new lesson. But for now, we need to be FTDI 100 percent. Pray for us!

Being mentally motivated to do what you ordinarily wouldn't want to do is critical in making change. It's all about the eating. The workouts are always challenging, but it's really about the food. We are both doing well, and now it's just about sticking to the plan. There are eleven days till my weigh-out. We decided today to eliminate carbs for the remainder of this week and into Monday December 7. We will also begin doing Calli tea on Sunday night.

Yesterday was a fun day because I officially fit into XL shirts. I have gone from 3XL to XL, my waist from 46 to 40. Although unofficial, my weight this morning was 258.5. My total weight loss to date is 43.4 pounds in just over eleven weeks. I bought a bunch of new clothes. My target for the end of this challenge weigh-out on December 14 is 247.0 pounds. I'm thinking 12 pounds in eleven days will do it.

There will be no workout tomorrow, but I'm going to resume on Saturday. It's going to be a test of staying focused on my goal, which is so close. Today I donated my old clothes to charity. It was amazing how much I donated. It also was sad because I had an emotional tie to some of those things. But it's out with the old and in with the new. It's exciting to be getting smaller, although I'm still big. But I'm no longer obese big. I feel good. I'm definitely healthier. I can now officially buy clothes in a regular store rather than just a big-and-tall store. This has never been the case for me.

Dressing well is expensive when you must shop at a big-and-tall store. Sure, there's more material being used, but there is also less competition, so you pay a premium. In some cases, brand names aren't even available. But not anymore! This is so cool. Skinny people just don't understand.

I also can't believe the cheerleaders we have. Social media is indeed awesome. A lot of people are enjoying our experience. Some need to join in for themselves, but they just aren't mentally ready. So many make a mini commitment after the holidays but then just fail, exactly as I have for thirty years. The problem is we so often take two steps forward and three back, ending up slightly bigger every year. Then twenty years go by, and we're a disaster. Unfortunately, sometimes things about our health are irreversible. I am so thankful that was not my case. I truly believe I can reverse all my bad health along with all my medications. I also look forward to never visiting my kidney doctor ever again, unless he wants to be a client of mine. Next week I'm going to eliminate all my medications, just in my final week, because of how radical my diet will be. I noticed eating no carbs is having a huge impact on my sugar levels, so I must eat a granola bar or something to pick up my sugar levels. I hoping this is just medication driven, so although I'm choosing to come off without consulting my doctor,

I will be closely monitoring my sugar levels and my blood pressure for the week. This should be interesting.

It's amazing! I have eliminated all seven of my medications. My sugar levels are in the 90s. My blood pressure was tested, and I was 96/68. This is clearly too low, but it is without medication. I'll keep checking my numbers, of course, but never since I was diagnosed with diabetes and high blood pressure have my numbers ever dropped to these levels.

We are officially in talapigus week. What does that mean? Well, all week our menu consists of tilapia and asparagus. Our tilapia is seasoned three ways, so there's a little bit of variety. In the beginning, this isn't so bad, but it does wear on you. We have some hazards coming up. Wednesday night we are attending a dinner at an Italian restaurant. Hopefully I can order just protein. But until then, stay focused.

It's Wednesday, and my workout went great in this final week. Tonight is the challenge. But at the same time, the old Mike Mendoza is saying, "I can't wait until tonight!"

Susie and I arrive at the restaurant. Mistake number one happens, and I order a drink. Then another. I justify because I order my Jack Daniels with Diet Coke. We sit for dinner but get no menus. Our host has selected the menu, and everything is being ordered family style. First the bread comes out, and I'm starving. I immediately morph back to the old Mike. Bread, butter, and OMG, this is so awesome. Salads are served—first a blue cheese wedge, my absolute favorite, then another salad, neither of which is FTDI. Continuously flowing food is hitting the table. Crab cakes, medallions of beef, calamari—it doesn't stop. Then pasta dishes. We are stuffed, and then come the desserts. I totally cave and consume everything as if it were my last supper. I leave feeling so great and at the same time so guilty. Tomorrow we have an all-day conference that ends in a luncheon. As of Wednesday night, I have four pounds to go.

I go through the next day really well. At the luncheon, which is buffet style, I stay away from all carbs, but the food choices aren't great. I don't know how much I have regressed, and just consume water the rest of the afternoon.

Friday I have a full day ahead of me. I take water and decide to hold out until having a late breakfast after my meeting. No carbs for breakfast! As I move through my Friday, I have nothing else but water. Dinner, I am back on talapigus.

I was not supposed to work out this final weekend, because I was not supposed to come off the talapigus, but I get up early and complete a seven o'clock workout. I feel I need it. I now have six pounds to lose by Monday morning. Susie packs me tilapia and asparagus with white rice in two containers because I will be gone most of the day. I start my morning with a protein shake and take only one of the containers. I'm going to cut my one meal into two. Protein shake, talapigus, protein shake, talapigus, with two and a half hours between each meal. I'm still drinking water but not as much. My day goes great, but there is some anxiety building because at this point I don't see any way I'm hitting my goal, and it's totally my fault.

Dinner comes, and it's talapigus with a little white rice again. By ten o'clock, I am absolutely starving. This is not the norm. I think my body is totally confused. I have nothing else. I am also getting sick now and have been on Nyquil at night and Dayquil by day. Susie tells me I need to limit my water intake.

On Sunday morning I weigh myself, and I have lost zero! I have six pounds to lose in twenty-four hours. How can this be possible? I'm feeling defeated and now very disappointed in myself. I am understanding I have very little self-control when in the wrong environment. I never realized how undisciplined I was when it came to food. It's so easy to say what I'm going to do. In the right environment, it really isn't that difficult. But when removed from the controlled environment at home or when Susie and I don't go to breakfast or lunch with an agenda, I am just a mess. One thing is for sure: I am learning a great deal about myself. My subconscious mind is overpowering my conscious mind. It's as if there is programming that overrides my conscious choices, and it's powerful.

I'm learning a little about neuro-linguistic programming (NLP), and I am understanding what is going on here. My mind has been programmed to be a fat person all my life, and now I'm trying to rewrite that program. My subconscious mind, I think, is interpreting my conscious mind as a virus and blocking the attempted change. I realize now what my next battle will be. Skinny people are programmed differently, so they have the reverse problem. They have to try to get fat, and it goes against their programming.

Now back to Sunday. I eat Egg Beaters with asparagus for breakfast. At noon I have my last meal of the day: the final tilapia-and-asparagus meal! At two o'clock it's Calli tea (dieters' tea) and no more water. By nine at night, this stuff is supposed to kick in and release everything I'm holding in my body. With six pounds to go, this will certainly have to be the crap of a lifetime.

Well, it's nine o'clock, and nothing. Susie tells me no Dayquil or Nyquil. I'm coughing and have a sore throat. No water, so I start taking sugar-free throat lozenges. They help tremendously. My mouth stays moist, and my cough is suppressed.

To stay distracted I'm watching TV, and it's now ten o'clock. The Calli tea has activated in Susie, and she's back and forth to the toilet. Me, nothing. It's now eleven, and I tell Susie to fix me another tea. She's a little concerned as to what the outcome may be, but I must do something. So I have another. Finally we are exhausted and go to bed at twelve thirty.

It's four in the morning, and shazam! I go running to the toilet excited and thankful. I won't go into the details, but it is remarkable. I can't believe what my body was holding back. Two flushes later I emerge from the bathroom and go back to bed. Unfortunately, I'm still coughing and have a sore throat. I'm not drinking water and am not sure how big an impact this has made on my weight. I am also not sure whether I will be heading back to the toilet soon, so I just lie there, unable to go back to sleep. My mind is all over the place. My weigh-in is 8:10 a.m. Part of me wishes it were later, to give me more time, and the other part wants to go reward myself with breakfast. Not a healthy one, of course. I know my body is dehydrated, and I know that before and after screwing up on Wednesday night, I did the best possible.

I get out of bed at seven. I go to the toilet, and nothing. It's as if I'm just totally empty. I stand on the scale, and I weigh 247. To win this challenge, I must weigh in on their scale below 247.3. My scale says 247, but it's not digitized, and I'm buck naked. Of course, I will need to be clothed when I weigh in. But I will tell you: I was amazed at the weight. I shave and shower. Susie is up and asks,

"Sooooo?" I tell her it's going to be close. I'm hoping for one more episode at the toilet because this is going to be a close one.

We head to the camp. Arriving, we must wait for them to call us. After about twenty minutes, we get called in. I take off my shirt, hoping it helps, but as I stand on the scale, I can see I'm not going to make it. I weigh in at 247.7. I miss my twenty pounds by four-tenths of a pound! It's easy to look back and say so many things to myself, but really I am proud of what I accomplished.

On September 14, I weighed in at 301.9. After my first six weeks, I weighed out of the first challenge at 267.3, down 34.6 pounds. I gained 11 pounds during my break—which was me being the old fat Mike, totally reverting back to who I was—and was behind at the start. On December 14, my final weight after the second challenge was 247.7, for a total weight loss of 54.2 pounds. I dropped from 3XL to XL. My waist went from 46 to 40, and those 40s are not snug. And even more important than all that, I am taking no medications.

Chapter 7

What's Next?

Clearly the story doesn't end here. When we are done with our challenge, we can do another, join for a year, or simply walk away. Susie is committed to staying on for the next year. I'm not, because the high impact has been really hard on me. But I want to because of the results I have had. I am a little concerned that if I revert back to what I used to do, I will become who I used to be. Joining this camp for the year is expensive, and more so because I didn't make my second challenge goal. They offer both Susie and me a discount of ten dollars per pound lost in the second challenge to join for the year. Without hesitation, I agree to pay for Susie, but I'm not committing myself yet. We are going to talk about it after leaving.

We go home, change, and head out to have that unhealthy breakfast. Then we are determined to go for dessert at Cinnabon. Now those are some great choices. While consuming three thousand–plus calories, we decide I should also join for the year. We have been workout partners for three months, and I enjoy doing this with her. We hold each other accountable. It won't be such an emotional roller coaster, because there is no longer a challenge and we know what we need to do. We have accepted we are going to screw up through the holidays, so we will just need to make more days good than bad. And we have both committed to being 100 percent back on FTDI right after the new year.

My ultimate goal was 240 pounds. Before breakfast I was just 7.7 pounds away. Susie still has a bunch more she wants to lose, so we are looking forward to our new goals. I am determined to hit the sixty-pound-total weight-loss goal and then learn to maintain that number for a while as I work on building back some muscle.

I realize there is still a lot of reprogramming that needs to be done with my mind, and I hope to achieve that over the next quarter. Being healthy and fit is a very difficult thing for fat people. We are just a few cheeseburgers and pizzas away from total relapse. But I think I must understand I can still have these things, just not every day.

Today is the beginning of a new journey. I am going to reintroduce myself to my old friends (those foods that are dangerous) while modifying how much and when I eat them. My clothes will be a good guideline, because all my old clothes are gone and I refuse to buy a larger size.

Tomorrow morning Susie and I will be back at the camp for our first workout as new members. I'm looking forward to it!

Weigh-out date was December 14. Fifty-four of my sixty goal pounds were lost. I feel great! I am wearing clothes I can buy in any store. I am just shy of my goal. My health is better than it has been in twenty years. My body feels a little beat up owing to the high impact, but everyone has noticed my weight loss. Compliments are continuously coming my way. I am talking to people about their health continuously. On social media I have a ton of fans, and people all over the country are asking me for information. I am so proud of myself!

As we approach the holidays, we are in the process of opening a new office. This is exciting and stressful. We're expending lots of money to do this, but we know we need to. This, combined with the holidays, combined with the workout routine, combined with my new healthier life, is a lot happening all at once.

It is Christmas time. Little by little our workout routine has become less consistent. Although we keep telling ourselves we must be careful with our food choices, we start to deviate. The problem is that nothing really seems to change much. Our clothes fit just fine, the compliments keep coming, and I'm feeling good. I'm checking my sugar levels and blood pressure, and everything is looking good. As Christmas approaches, we start the move to our new office. It is becoming very stressful, but we know that right after Christmas we have planned a trip to Las Vegas to ring in the new year. This will be the ultimate stress reliever.

Even though I'm not making consistently good food choices, I am not noticing size gain. My clothes are all fitting fine, and I am slowing taking my eye off the ball, as if I had a disease before but now I'm cured. I'm conscious of my health, but it is not a priority, where just a month ago, it was my top priority.

We get through Christmas and officially move into our new office before the new year and head to Las Vegas. The plan is to have as much fun as possible and ring in the new year. It is our anniversary, it's a new chapter in our lives, we have new bodies, and we are healthier than ever. Right after we get home, we are going to get after it again and hit our final goals!

It doesn't matter what we eat or drink. We know this time right now is just temporary, and we already know what we need to do to get back on track. We have a clear, precise meal plan. We are now full members of our boot camp. We have made a ton of friends at our boot camp, who keep cheering us on.

It is impossible to fail. Our final goals will be achieved, and we will then continue on to maintenance. I will finish this short book with such a great story of overcoming what seemed to be impossible but is indeed possible for anyone who will just make a commitment. But there is one problem: I forgot I am a fat person.

Just because I lost all this weight, it didn't change who I am. It just changed who I have temporarily become. I like who I have become, but I don't like the things I had to do to arrive to that point.

I have never come down this path before, at least to this extent. I have gone on hundreds of diets, losing weight and gradually gaining it all back plus more. I think to myself, "Going on a diet is bad, because each time I stop, I gain back not only my weight but more."

I even stop writing this book. I think it's over, and I just need a happy ending. But at this moment it's May 2. Five months have passed.

Paul Simon wrote a song many years ago called "Slip Slidin' Away." It a great song to listen to and one that applies as we close this chapter.

CHAPTER 8

The Relapse

As I stated at the end of the last chapter, it's five months later. What I thought was the end of the book was not at all. I am a fat person. This is not common sense. A friend of mine, Chuck, says in our business accountability meeting that we all know what we need to do on a daily basis. He uses the analogy of weight loss and says, "You want to lose weight. In front of you are a salad and a cheeseburger. Which should you pick? It's easy! So the same goes with your business." That analogy is so logical. But it came from a skinny person! And skinny people don't understand. It is not logical.

I was told I am a type 2 diabetic. I was told once a diabetic, always a diabetic. I am just now a diabetic that doesn't need all that medication. It is being controlled by diet. But I will always be a diabetic. Well, likewise, I am a fat person. I will always be a fat person. It will just have to be controlled by diet. I really think that sucks! It's not fair! Why can't I be like those skinny people with a racing metabolism who can eat everything they want and never gain any weight? Well, I don't know why. And most of you reading this book know exactly how I feel. But we aren't those people. We are us. Call us Team Fatso!

I start not to fit so well in my old clothes. In fact, some things stop fitting altogether. From New Year's to the beginning of April, I become the old me again. I step on a scale to see how bad things have gotten. I didn't gain ten, fifteen, or even twenty pounds. I gained over thirty from my low. I did build back some muscle, but along with that I also gained back inches I had lost. It is evident in my clothes.

During this time, we travel quite a bit, going in February to the Atlantis Resort in the Bahamas, which is awesome. We go to Florida twice. Susie is also in Louisiana. In March, we are in Maui. My mother-in-law, who was living with us and being cared for by us, dies. This lady lived to be ninety-three and a half. What an incredible life-span. But it is nonetheless a difficult emotional time for the entire family, so we leave to Maui to escape.

Would it be possible to continue to eat healthy during all this? Of course, but I'm a fat person, and that's not how we roll! What was mutually agreed on was we would eat FTDI 90 percent of the time and 10 percent of the time we could mess up. What really happens is we gradually work our way to the opposite. Our workouts are here and there but not consistent. The conscious thought is there, but the necessary choices are not.

Because the effects are very slow, they creep up. People say you lose all that weight, and then you have one bad meal and gain it back. Well, that's not true. It takes a lot of bad meals.

I do not wish bad health on anyone. You could very well be overweight or morbidly obese, which I was, but you might not suffer from high blood pressure, high triglycerides, high cholesterol, or type 2 diabetes, as I do. In my case, high blood pressure was my blessing. It was my alarm clock.

As April approaches—you know that month, tax-filing deadline month—I start to have faint headaches. Not consistent but kind of like pressure. They come and go. I don't think much about them. Susie and I decide we must get back on track. Even more so for me, because my clothes aren't fitting, which in itself is an alarm clock. Going back to the market and buying the right foods is the beginning. It doesn't mean we are going to eat right every day, but we are heading in the right direction. Eating out in restaurants is the worst thing we can do. We think we make fairly good choices, but really there aren't very many good choices eating out. Even those that seem to be healthy can be worse than just a cheeseburger or pasta.

Those faint headaches are becoming more frequent, but they're not much more than a little annoying. Then, on April 22, I go in for a routine visit with my regular doctor. I have been very conscious of my eating and have been working out for about ten days before this so I wouldn't go in with obvious problems (accountability). First thing, they weigh me. I am very unhappy with myself. I am letting myself down. Then they check my blood pressure, which I stopped checking for months, even though I know I am supposed to. I didn't, because after my weight loss, I tricked myself into believing I had cured my disease and it was no longer necessary.

My blood pressure is 205/105. The doctor tells me, "I would rather see you in the ER rather than my office with these numbers." He says, "I'm going to give you some medication, and if your blood pressure doesn't come down, you will have to be admitted into the hospital." *Crap!* Talk about an alarm clock. Even though I made an attempt to get better before this appointment, I didn't. Those faint headaches were actually becoming stronger. My blood pressure comes down with the medication, and I am able to leave the doctor's office.

On Friday night we go to a movie. My head is now just a continuous annoyance. I now am thinking, "What have I done to myself? I was given the opportunity to continue my life in great health, and I blew it." The whole time we're in the movie, *The Jungle Book*, I am not right. I am not feeling right physically. I have a great deal of anxiety, and I tell myself, "I have to fix this immediately or go back to my kidney doctor and tell him I need more medication." This is actually what my regular internist said I needed to do immediately. I tell myself, "Hang in there one week, and let's see what happens."

On Saturday I have a training session at my office. I am 100 percent focused on what I know I should be doing with eating and drinking a ton of water. After training I attend a nonprofit event, and that evening we go to a graduation party. My head now is hurting more than Friday, and even though I'm trying to mask my feelings, Susie knows I'm not right. I don't want her to be concerned about me, because she is still grieving the loss of her mother.

On Sunday I'm feeling a little better, but not great. We are having a potluck for our team. I know I'm going to eat poorly and drink, but I am going to limit myself on everything and remember to drink a bunch of water.

On Monday I'm back at the camp and committed to staying FTDI. I know this week is an all-out change back to what I know I'm supposed to be doing—or back to the doctor for medication if my body doesn't get fixed.

Here's what happens with my blood pressure:

Monday	190/108
Tuesday	166/84
Wednesday	152/91 (headaches gone)
Thursday	146/74
Friday	137/78

My sugar levels are fine. I tested at 119 blood glucose level. I'm down six pounds!

My body has responded well. I now know what I must do. In two weeks I'm traveling again: this time to New York for my birthday.

Chapter 9

Time Heals All Wounds (Not True)

WHAT SKINNY PEOPLE don't understand is that fat people don't get it. It's not so easy. This chapter is dedicated to all the people who know and understand my life. This chapter starts a year after chapter 7. Susie said to me yesterday, "I'm pathetic and I'm fat!" My reply was, "You're not pathetic."

As time has moved on, I have completely reverted back to the old me in every way. My weight loss is zero again. What is it really? Three hundred pounds. We have had a great year of traveling and eating. Well, inch by inch it was a cinch to as I added those inches and pounds back on. I have with great ease, gained back that weight that was so hard to work off.

Susie is not happy and says she wants to start over and do a new challenge. I tell her I can't. When we went back to our boot camp, my knees were killing me, so my solution has been not to work out. Now my knees are killing me even without workouts. Everything in life is great except my health.

I must go back to the doctor, but I do blood tests first. What was I expecting when I visited with my doctor? To be scolded. My blood pressure is 188/100—not good. My A1C is 8.1—not good. I am spilling record amounts of protein into my urine—not good. But I feel great! Not really. What I have learned is my body adapts and how I feel isn't how I am.

We just got back from a trip to Orlando. We went for Valentine's week and went to be kids again. We had a great time; however, my knees were killing me. I had to endure pain the entire trip. That really sucks. I saw people on those motorized carts and thought, "That's really a good idea. I should get one of those." But that would be the beginning of the end.

We both come back frustrated about our weight. Susie officially rejoins the camp to start a new challenge. I can't physically handle the workouts, so I am going to follow the eating plan and go to Camp Snoopy (my regular gym).

I am going to track my progress and must succeed at and maintain this, because there may never another time. I am going to be thirty again. Most people get to be thirty twice in their lives, but few get to do it three times, as my mother-in-law did. It's hard for me to accept I am going to become sixty years old. Old people are sixty years old. You can now take retirement money without penalty at sixty years old. Noooooo! I'm just going to be thirty again!

I am three hundred pounds and motivated to do this again. I remember what it felt like over a year ago when I came off my second challenge. I remember how great it felt to wear XL shirts and sweaters and pants that I didn't remember fitting into for thirty years. I remember fifty-four pounds ago.

I remember how happy Susie was at her lower weight too. I bought her new clothes. I bought myself new clothes. We got nothing but compliments from people. All those cheerleaders! And they were cheering us not because we were special but just because we became normal. Not because we were skinny but because we were no longer obese. I remember coming off my medications for a brief moment and my doctor being amazed with my accomplishment.

This is not a six-week or twelve-week challenge. This is a life challenge. That's where the real fear is!

Pray for me! Round 2 begins now! It is Sunday, and as we dieters do, I plan to begin changing on Monday. How many times have we said this?

Skinny people absolutely do not understand!

CHAPTER 10

Live to Eat or Eat to Live

I THINK PEOPLE like us either just throw in the towel and give up or make the choice to change. I, like so many others, am diabetic and have high blood pressure. Fortunately, I have no signs of permanent damage, and I believe that my situation is reversible.

Having been in the financial industry for twenty-three years now, I have visited with thousands of people setting up life insurance plans and investment accounts. When I look at the statistics, 54 percent of all people end up dependent on family or the government by age sixty-five. Thirty-six percent are still working, mostly because they have to. Five percent have died. Four percent are OK, and 1 percent are wealthy. Of those 95 percent that remain living, 50 percent will die before age eighty-five. Of that remaining group, only about 5 percent will continue on to age ninety.

As for me, I really don't want to be part of the 5 percent that doesn't make it to sixty-five. In fact, I don't want to die before eighty-five either. I have some money invested. Maybe I won't be in the wealthy 1 percent, but I know I will be OK financially.

When it comes to retirement, there are three phases we go through:

Go-go phase: We are active and very mobile, going after the bucket list, revisiting the areas we enjoyed in our lives.

Slow-go phase: We go on cruises, go to casinos, visit grandkids, and remember to take our medications.

No-go phase: We stay home, and now people visit us or take us places.

What's important to me is not just living beyond eighty-five but also hanging on to that go-go phase as long as I can. Maybe I had to get this old before really understanding this.

I do believe the consistency of working out and retaining a gym membership for many years has helped. I have yo-yo dieted all my life, but the continuous activity, in spite of me being morbidly obese, has helped me not to have permanent damage. Also, visiting my doctor and temporarily heeding his or her advice to lose weight and never neglecting to take any prescribed medications have been factors.

So week 1 begins with 100 percent FTDI. How is it? Awful! But at the end of week 1, I have dropped ten pounds. More importantly, my blood pressure has gone from 182/101 to 134/73. My blood sugar has gone from 183 to 94. Obviously, I am pushing my limits at just ten pounds heavier.

Also, I can fit into my clothes correctly and am noticeably more comfortable. This point right here is where most of us begin to quit our diets! I caught myself thinking that way. It is truly a mental thing!

The difference here is I am not in the boot camp. I am not being held accountable as I was the first time. I am accountable only to myself. I have created a weekly chart to monitor myself. It's on my computer desktop, and it's printed and taped to my door to see every day. I have set goals I believe are realistic. I am drinking a lot of water. I mean *a lot* of water. At the same time, I'm experimenting with high-alkaline water (pH over 8) to see how it affects me. There's lots of hype on this, and I'm not sold on it yet. I will give it two to three weeks and let you know my thoughts, because it is expensive compared to spring water, which is what I normally drink.

Susie joined the boot camp, but after ten days, she has to stop because she had a pain in her lower abdomen. The doctor says she has to get a CT scan and orders her to stop working out.

Going into the second week, we aren't off FTDI, but we are modifying it and doing a lot of research. After my second week, I have lost only one pound, but my blood pressure remains normal, and my sugar levels are below normal. I am given an additional medication for my diabetes, and the goal is to stop it in about a week and see how I respond.

Week 3 we remain on a modified FTDI plan but are talking about paleo. Again, it's a bunch of hype, and we don't know whether it will work for us, but we may make the switch. For me, the paleo diet may be easier to follow. Maybe it's just a guy thing.

What FTDI and paleo have in common is that both eliminate sugars and processed foods. Both require lots of water. Both are dairy-free. Both include no legumes (beans). Both include no bread or flour or corn tortillas or chips. Both include no white or russet potatoes. These are the things embedded in our diets that are bad, bad, bad for us non-skinny people. But we crave them so, so much. These are the things we will battle the most to eliminate. Skinny people will say, "But it's OK once in a while," because they don't understand. It's like telling an alcoholic it's OK to have occasional drinks.

We all must find our own ways through this struggle. We must wage a war of not allowing ourselves to eat out. We must fight off all the marketing on TV, radio, billboards, and social media about the foods we desire so much but can't have because they're killing us. This is an extremely hard battle, and skinny people don't understand. We aren't the ones who desire and order a kale salad or quinoa as a side dish to our salmon. We don't ask for the dressing on the side or hold the this or that. We want it all with butter and bacon!

You, my friend, understand me. For breakfast we may order oatmeal, but we want the eggs, bacon, home fries, and waffles or french toast. We justify our pancakes because we have fruit on them, and then we have coffee with Splenda. We drink Diet Coke because we think it cancels something else out. We wear sweatpants because they are comfortable, not because we actually plan on sweating.

OK, back to this diet stuff. The rant is over. Let's compare FTDI to Paleo, and maybe this will help you should you decide to take this journey with me.

FTDI Diet

Proteins:
Meat: chicken breast, turkey breast, and extra-lean ground turkey
Fish: tilapia and tuna
Eggs: egg whites or Egg Beaters

Protein shakes (stay under 140 calories)

Vegetables: broccoli, spinach, asparagus, kale, and brussels sprouts

Carbs: brown rice, quinoa, and oatmeal

Spices OK, avoid salt
Sweeteners: no sugar, avoid artificial sweeteners, stevia OK

Instructions: Eat a meal every two and a half hours. A protein shake counts as a meal. Alternate protein shake and food meals, eating six times a day. Drink a minimum of one gallon of water daily.

Paleo Diet

Proteins:
Meats, fish, and eggs (Grass-fed beef is preferable. Be cautious of the quality of all meats or fish. Eggs are best if cage-free, pasture raised, and scratch fed.)

Carbs: plantains, yams, sweet potatoes, cassava (raw), taro root, carrots, butternut squash, spaghetti squash, and pumpkin

Vegetables: no limits if green, eat lots of color, only moderation or limits on starchy vegetables

Fruits: portion control but should be included daily; berries are the best choice; apples, pears, bananas, citrus, and so on; and yes, avocados

Nuts and seeds: eat in moderation, but they're acceptable (I didn't know, but peanuts and cashews are not nuts; they are legumes.)

What's important with these foods is serving sizes. You can't just eat all you want of all approved foods, except for vegetables. There seems to be no limit for vegetables, but make sure what you believe is a vegetable is actually a vegetable and not a fruit or root or legume.

Whatever you select as your meal plan, stick with it for a while, and see whether it's working for you. For us with eating disorders, no diet is something we get excited about. It's never going to be. When you are committing to a diet, you become excited to reach your goal so you can go onto maintenance. You know that part: when we can now go back to eating what we want but in "moderation."

We will cover maintenance later, because that's where I have always failed.

CHAPTER 11

Eat like a Caveman

WE MUST ALL find our own ways to what works, and most importantly it must be sustainable. We have officially made the switch to paleo. I say "we" because I rely so much on Susie and she has been the one reading and understanding this diet. She is following a guy named Robb Wolf. We also have a nephew and his wife who have been on paleo for a really long time and stuck to it. Susie reads and inquires, and then she gives me the Cliffs Notes. All I need to know is what's OK and not OK to eat and keep it simple. I'm two weeks into this, and I can live with it.

I give up all grains and anything made with grains. Yes, that means breads, cakes, donuts, tortillas, cereals, bagels, pancakes, waffles, french toast, pastas, and beer. No rice, corn, or beans of any kind, which includes peanuts and cashews, which are legumes, or anything that contains these things. No artificial sweeteners of any kind. No sugars, but I can use stevia (not Truvia). No dairy, whether it be milk, ice cream, or cheese. No processed foods of any kind. No canola oil or any oils that are processed.

Pretty much everything else is on the good list! I can have free-range eggs, uncured bacon, uncured ham, grass-fed beef, and free-range chicken and turkey. Pork, all parts, is good so long as it is not processed and has no added sulfates. Fish and seafood are all good to go! The oils that are OK to use are olive, coconut, and avocado. I can also use ghee. I never heard of this until now, but it is a class of clarified butter. Fruit is OK in moderation, as well as all vegetables. On the potato side, sweet potatoes are the best option, but those russets that we have grown to love are off the table.

Although I am going on only my third week, I have been losing weight. The last ten days I haven't been working out, because I have been sick with the flu. But today I go back to the gym. From starting with the FTDI diet, which I was finding difficult maintaining, to making the paleo switch, I am down a total of twenty pounds. All my numbers—blood pressure and sugars—are in the normal range, and more importantly, I have eliminated the added medication given to me thirty days ago for my diabetes.

So I'm beginning a new lifestyle on the paleo (Paleolithic) diet.

So back to the present. Things are moving along, and we are invited to a dinner event at the Old Spaghetti Factory. The meal choices were selected for us ahead of an evening training. Here's what I am learning: stay away from eating out in an uncontrolled environment, which is called a restaurant. We don't have the willpower to make good choices, and worse, in this case, the limited choices are all bad.

The truth of the meal is this: I select chicken marsala. It is the best worst choice. While eating the meal, I get a tingling sensation in my mouth, tongue, and lips. I don't know whether it is the sodium or what, but its entry into my body is not good. My body knows this is not good for me. How do I respond? I eat it all anyway. But it is a clear sign: the food we eat in restaurants is poisoning us. When you are eating clean and away from it, the body knows. This is a good lesson.

I have found that when I mess up, I seem to continue, like an alcoholic falling off the wagon. I know that I'm messing up every few meals, but I have a hard time getting back on track.

I love bread and butter. I can eat warm bread until people stop bringing it to me, even though I know it's not good to eat. Grains in general cause inflammation, which is something else I fight. I enjoy eating cereal as well, even what is viewed as "healthy" cereal. But there still remains that grain-and-inflammation thing. I don't have a gluten problem, but I do retain water.

As we fast-forward through the year, I am on and off paleo. I have added magnesium and turmeric supplements to my diet. These were recommended for my high blood pressure and inflammation. When I'm off it, I can feel it. I get back on, and I feel and sleep better. Then out of nowhere, I get a pain in my hip. My solution: go to the gym and work it out. Worst thing I could have done.

Day by day the pain gets worse. It intensifies just before I am ready to go on four consecutive weeks of travel. I am having trouble even sleeping. While I'm in Dallas to visit my kids, it is the worst. I have to sleep in a chair. I am given medications, hydrocodone and Flexeril and a few others, but nothing helps except alcohol. I now understand real pain, which is nothing I have ever had to endure in my life!

After getting back from my last trip, I get an MRI. It is determined I have moderate to severe spinal stenosis in my L4 and L5. A nerve is being pinched by my vertebrae, causing pain from my hip all the way to my ankle. In this same sequence of events, I also go to see an orthopedic doctor, who I had previously scheduled to reevaluate my ankle, which was diagnosed as having crushed cartilage back in July 2014. Turns out I was misdiagnosed and wearing an ankle brace was the worst thing I could have done for the last three years.

So what proceeds is physical therapy. Stretching, stretching, and more stretching. After six weeks of physical therapy and stretching at home, I'm feeling like the old me. Then my knees start hurting! This has been a problem for years, but I guess the other pains just canceled the knee pain. *Pain sucks.*

I go to the Los Angeles county fair. I have sore knees and still some pain in my ankle. I'm having a great time, but walking a lot gets painful. At the fair are creams and lotions and electrical devices that will supposedly eliminate every pain I have, but they all look like gimmicks to me. Then I see this vibration platform. It looks like a doctor's scale and reminds me of the Footsie Wootsie I bought years back, which has always comforted my feet with high-speed vibration. With my ankles and knees hurting, I decide to hop on. I stay on because it feels great. After ten minutes, I get off. My knees no longer hurt, and I feel no pain in my ankle. I ask the guy what the price is, and it is ridiculous. I walk away.

I continue to walk through the fair, and I tell Susie I feel so much better. Then, a few aisles down, I find another booth that has a similar machine, which looks more like one I would find in a doctor's office. I get on, and the guy shows me how I should use it and tells me about the physical benefits of using it daily. All I know is I feel better. What is that worth? So I ask, "How much?" He says it's $999, which is $2,000 less than the other guy. So I buy it.

It's been just a couple of weeks, and I'm still very cautious with all my movements because of all I have been through, but I am no longer walking with a limp, and my knees are no longer hurting. Best $1,000 I could have spent!

Chapter 12

The Search for What Works

We all must face it, and getting old sucks. When we are young, we can get away with eating anything. Very few of us think of our health. Those of us who are fat or will begin the process of becoming fat in our early years figure out how to enjoy everything that is bad for our health but tastes great. This will later affect not only our weight and size but also our health and mobility. Those who remain unaware end up taking a bunch of medications and later have a walker or even a wheelchair or motorized cart. For many, this happens far too early in life.

For those of us who are aware, we start fighting the battle early on. Maybe around thirty-five or forty, we realize there is a problem. We go on diets and go to the gym, but for most of us, we are already addicted to the bad habits. So we yo-yo. We support every gym and fitness center out there. We are the reason Weight Watchers, Jenny Craig, Nutrisystem, Lindora, Herbalife, and countless others exist. We all are trying to find an easy fix, a magic pill or medical treatment that's going to make us "normal." Then, in that process, fighting that battle, we get *old*.

Now I think, "F———, I'm sixty!" Through my eyes, looking at the world, I still see young—as long as I don't look in the mirror. I could say the pains are from age, but I don't think so. So I'm not giving up!

As I come to the end of this writing, I am concluding that the paleo diet is what's best for me. Not eating grains, combined with the turmeric, has eliminated my inflammation, which also contributes to pain. Greatly reducing sugars and carbs in my diet has reduced my glucose levels, therefore helping me control my diabetes. Remaining paleo most of the time, I feel better and sleep better. When I totally blow it and head to Krispy Kreme or have that giant cinnamon roll or have a candy or ice-cream binge, I know it can be just that moment, and then I've got to get back on paleo and stay away from eating out.

The vibration therapy is working for me. I am continually stretching and maintain a daily awareness of my body and how I feel. I enjoy cardio and the sweat that comes with it, but I'm very cautious with what I do, because I don't want to injure my body. I have learned that high-intensity workouts are not my solution but rather increase my chances of injury.

This is my life, and skinny people don't understand. Skinny people will never understand, and I'm OK with it. What's really important is I understand. I must understand me, and I must have the continual desire to want to live an enjoyable life with movement, free of pain, as long as I can.

Maintenance is our hell. We don't comprehend moderation. We lose weight and are happy with the way we look. We are happy with the way we feel. But we are not happy enough that we maintain. Why? Maybe because we no longer get any recognition.

When we don't understand something, what should we do? Well, I Googled it. One of the articles said, "To maintain weight loss, you are essentially fighting a system that's wired to regain lost pounds."

So that's it! It's not my fault; it's my body's fault. And we need to blame someone other than ourselves. Sounds like every article I read is written by a skinny person. So here is my non-PhD, non-nutritionist, nonprofessional answer: We don't maintain weight loss, simply because it isn't important enough to maintain weight loss. We are eating alcoholics. We need support groups and don't have any. All the diets and weight-loss methods are out there, and all we fat folks buy into them. And even if we follow them, we don't get a chip for one month or one year or five years "sober." We are all on our own. We get attention for losing the weight, and then it fades away. We don't have new goals when it comes to weight loss.

But you know what? Cigarette smokers are addicted to nicotine. So how do they quit and never go back? They simply never want to smoke again badly enough. They may be our best counselors. So here are some ideas to help you through the toughest stage of your weight struggle, as taught to cigarette smokers:

1. Keep a list of the reasons you must maintain your weight loss. Look at that list every day.

2. Build a support system. Surround yourself with people who want you to succeed in maintaining your weight loss. As soon as you start your diet, tell your friends and family. The more people you tell you need support in this difficult task in your life, the harder it will be for you to just give up and relapse.

3. Exercise no fewer than five times a week. Even if you can't get to a gym, go for walks, and keep moving. "I'm tired" is not acceptable.

4. Buy a calendar. At the end of every day, mark a big red X on that day if you ate correctly. When you see continuous progress, pat yourself on the back for doing such a great job.

5. Reward yourself. Celebrate small victories. Treat yourself to a movie or a sporting event. Buy a new outfit.

6. Don't let yourself rationalize eating poorly, even if just one day. And if it seems hopeless or you are in a really bad environment, make the best "bad" choices you can. And don't listen to the demons in your life that are not supportive and tell you it's OK to have a couple of donuts, an ice-cream sundae, cake, or whatever will get you to fall off the wagon. They don't understand if they are skinny, or fat friends who want to bring you back to their world.

7. Focus on the advantages of your weight loss continuously. Keep reminding yourself about how great you look and how great you feel. It is a battle of you against you. Never think about what you are missing out on because you shouldn't eat it, but rather how you are benefiting from staying away from it.

8. Believe in yourself! Think back to what you have accomplished. Every day you avoid making bad food choices is a victory. Most everybody gives up, but that's not you!

Writing this book is my self-help. I want to find the best way to help myself, and I pray that finding my way helps you find yours.

We must make two commitments before we start:

1. We must commit to doing whatever it takes to shed the weight. While doing so, we must clearly understand that skinny people don't understand what we will be or are actively going through. We cannot listen to skinny people. We should just graciously accept their compliments.
2. We must commit to fighting the never-ending battle of maintaining that weight loss we fought so hard to achieve—again, understanding that skinny people don't and never will understand the battle we live with.

We are special and unique people. We need to learn to love ourselves and do the best we can to keep ourselves alive and healthy for as long as we can. Our battle is forever, and we must accept that.

Hitting a weight goal for us is not the finish line. It is indeed an achievement, but cannot ever be confused with being that finish line. That weight goal is simply the beginning of a life long battle to maintain. We will have failures during our time of maintaining, but we must remind ourselves we must get back to the right choices quickly. It is too easy to slip slide away.

I pray for you and ask you pray for me through this journey of life.

About the Author

Michael J. Mendoza has struggled with his weight all his life and has written a book for others who face similar challenges.

Mendoza is a lifelong resident of Southern California. He earned his bachelor's degree in business accounting and now works as a financial adviser and business owner.